D0963696

liquididea press

Slow Carb
Fat Loss

Fast Fat Loss with the Slow Carb Diet

liquididea press

Keywords: slow carb, fat loss, liquididea press, diet, weight loss, slow carb diet, 4-hour body, dieting

Contents

Introduction..1

The Basics..3

PAGG Supplementation 9

Bingeing (a.k.a. Cheat Day)...11

Cheat Sheet 14

Cheat Sheet Frequently Asked Questions.......................16

Shopping List 19

Meal Plan #1...21

Meal Plan #2...25

Effectiveness of Slow Carb / Fat Loss Regimen..............33

Why Calories-In/Calories-Out is a Fallacy......................37

If It's Not Working..41

Taking a Cold Shower 43

Cut Outs 45

Acknowledgements 57

Introduction

In December 2011, I bought a copy of Tim Ferriss's *The 4-Hour Body*. Starting the day after Christmas, I eagerly devoured it, starting on a path that would lead to me to lose weight and increase my fitness and well-being.

The 4-Hour Body (or 4HB) became an overnight bestseller, hitting #1 on the *New York Times* Best Seller list, and inspiring millions to change their lives for the better.

I loved the book, as well, buying copies for friends and family and telling everyone I could about it.

As great as the 4HB is, it does have a few small shortcomings. On my first reading, I noticed that the otherwise excellent book lacked any summary of the many dozens of suggestions it made. The more I read the reference tome (it is 592 pages), the more I found myself flipping back and forth. And as the days passed, I found myself struggling to remember what to do when.

So I created a 4-Hour Body fat loss "cheat sheet" -- a one page summary of what to do when. It was just for my personal use, but then I thought to post it on my blog at williamhertling.com. This cheat sheet quickly became my highest volume article, racking up thousands of views per day.

I continued to write blog posts about *The 4-Hour Body*, specifically focused on the first quarter of the book: the fat loss regimen. These posts, which included example meal plans, recipes, a shopping list, how-to articles on taking a cold shower or doing exercises became my most popular posts, eventually bringing hundreds of thousands of readers to my site.

Even though I had already consolidated spread out information and supplemented missing information, I still received feedback from readers asking for more. In particular, they wanted me to take the tips and supplementary information spread out across a dozen blog posts and package that all neatly together into a single, simple to use booklet.

The result of that work is in your hands today. I hope this book makes your journey to fat loss and body recomposition using the slow carb diet successful and easier.

Please note that this booklet is not intended as a replacement for reading *The 4-Hour Body*. Please do buy a copy and read it. (I own two copies, and I've bought more for friends and family.) It's well worth the price, and it's the only way to understand why to do what Tim recommends.

The purpose of this book is only to consolidate small subsets of information together in a convenient, smaller form factor. Also, this book focuses only on the fat loss section (the slow carb diet, supplements, and exercises), a small fraction of Tim's shared wisdom.

Like Tim says, it would be really sad if you were injured or died. Use common sense, consult with a medical professional as needed, and don't do anything in this book, *The 4-Hour Body*, or anything else you read or watch without carefully understanding it.

Good luck,
William Hertling
Liquididea Press

The Basics

Tim Ferriss explains the principles of *The 4-Hour Body*, the slow carb diet, and the fat loss regimen beautifully and at length in *The 4-Hour Body*. I highly recommend it.

Here's my take on a quick recap of the key principles of the slow carb diet and related activities.

1. Avoid White Foods

Sugars, starches, grains - any food that is white or can be white - must be avoided.

Eating these types of foods, which are sugars or are quickly converted to sugars in the body, increases blood sugar levels. As blood sugar levels increase, insulin increases. Insulin is a hormone that helps move sugar from the blood into fat cells for long-term storage.

This has two negative effects. First, it contributes to fat gain as the extra calories are stored in fat cells. Second, it creates a roller-coaster effect: blood sugar levels spike rapidly after we consume carbohydrate rich foods, which causes insulin levels to spike in response, which lowers blood sugar levels to the point where we feel lethargic. This prompts us to eat more sugary food to regain our energy level.

Within a few days of starting the slow carb diet I began to feel as though I had more energy throughout the day, without any periods where I felt drained. This is one of the benefits that many 4HB practitioners relate experiencing.

The only types of carbohydrates that the 4HB recommends eating are vegetables and legumes, both of which contain abundant amounts of dietary fiber.

This means no: sugar, soda (including diet soda), wheat, bread, potatoes, dairy products (butter is OK since it is mostly fat).

2. Eat Sufficient Protein

Protein helps keep up our metabolic consumption, helps increase our feeling of satiation (we feel less hungry), spreads out the energy we get over a longer period of time, and contains less useable calories per gram than either carbohydrates or fats.

The amount of protein may be surprising. Tim recommends 30 grams of protein at breakfast and at least 20 grams at lunch and dinner. (More if you get hungry between meals.)

This doesn't mean consuming 30 grams of a protein-rich food, like chicken. It means 30 net grams of protein itself. Research the nutritional breakdown of the foods you eat to get an idea of how much you'll need to obtain this amount of protein.

For example, searching for "chicken nutrition" in Google helped me discover that 140 grams of chicken (no skin, just white meat) contains 43 grams of protein. There are about 28 grams per ounce, so it requires eating about five ounces of chicken breast to obtain 43 grams of protein.

This level of calorie counting and analysis isn't necessary on a regular basis for the Slow Carb diet (in fact, Tim recommends against it), but it is helpful to initially establish the approximate levels of protein sources you'll need to eat.

3. Every Meal Consists of Protein, Vegetables and Legumes

If meals don't include carbohydrates, what should they look like? According to Tim Ferriss, every meal should include protein, vegetables, and legumes.

As mentioned above, Tim recommends at least thirty grams of protein at breakfast to kick-start your metabolism. This can be accomplished, for example, by having three eggs plus some legumes. Other meals should include at least twenty grams of protein. Proteins that Tim recommends are: *egg whites with 1-2 whole eggs, *chicken breast or thigh, beef, fish, pork

Legumes should be about a half cup serving. Some recommended ones are: lentils, *black beans, pinto beans, red beans, soybeans.

Vegetables should be as much as desired. As Tim says, it takes a lot of spinach to equal even a small amount of calories. Some recommended options are: *Spinach, *Mixed vegetables (inc. broccoli, cauliflower, or other cruciferous), *Sauerkraut, *Kimchee, Peas, Green Beans, etc.

* These are associated with the fastest fat loss in his experience.

In my opinion, refried black beans are a great option that goes well with eggs.

4. Eat Simple, Repetitive Meals

Having simple, repetitive meals is a cornerstone of successful dieting. It's a simple fact that when we taste a novel, delicious dish, we'll eat more of it. Boring, in this case, is an advantage. In 4HB, Tim says "Pick three or four meals and repeat them."

5. Eat Meals, Not Snacks

Snack foods, even relatively healthy snack foods like nuts, are trouble foods (domino foods in 4HB speak) because we can just keep on consuming them. Tim draws the analogy that even a potato chip would be fine to eat if you could eat just one, but nobody can.

To counter-act this effect, eat meals, not snacks. If you are legitimately hungry before the next meal (not merely eating out of habit or boredom), then increase your meal size accordingly.

In my personal experience, I will allow myself a shot-glass size serving of nuts between meals if I am exceptionally hungry or in maintenance-mode, as opposed to full-on weight loss.

6. Don't Drink Calories

You may have as much water as you want, and as much unsweetened tea or coffee as you like. But don't drink milk, milk alternatives, sodas, or fruit juice. (Even diet soda has been strongly associated with weight gain[1].)

Tim has one glass of red wine before bed, and recommends red wine over white wine for fat loss.

Personally, I had one hard alcohol drink per night, and still feel I was successful in achieving my weight goals.

7. Don't Eat Fruit

Tim recommends in 4HB that you do not eat fruit. As he relates, in most parts of the world, people do not have access to fruit year-round. For example Europeans wouldn't be eating fruit during the winter. So the slow carb diet does not have fruit six days a week. (You can eat it on cheat day, of course.)

Personally, I eat fruit a few days a week during the summer season, as I'm not going to pass up the chance at fresh berries and figs when they are seasonally available. But as Tim says, that's only a limited portion of the year. The rest of the year, I can do without, while I get what I need nutritionally from vegetables.

8. Take One Day Off Per Week

According to *The 4-Hour Body*, if our bodies remain on a restricted diet for too long, it's possible for our metabolic rate to decrease. To counteract that effect, and to help maintain compliance the rest of the time, Tim Ferriss

---

[1] http://www.cbsnews.com/8301-504763_162-20075358-10391704/new-study-is-wake-up-call-for-diet-soda-drinkers/

recommends that one day a week should be a binge day. Anything goes! We can and should eat as much as we want, of anything we want.

If you want to eat pie and ice cream all day, you can. That being said, Tim does make specific recommendations about how to have the most successful cheat day in *The 4-Hour Body* that you should follow. These tips are summarized in the Cheat Day section.

PAGG Supplementation

Tim Ferriss recommends a combination of four supplements to enhance fat loss. PAGG is an acronym for:
Policosanol (20-25mg)
Alpha-lipoic acid (100-300mg)
Green tea flavanols (decaffeinated, 325mg EGCG)
Garlic extract (200mg)

Tim recommends PAGG before meals and bed for the following schedule:
Before breakfast: AGG
Before lunch: AGG
Before dinner: AGG
Before bed: PA(G)G

Some people that suffer from insomnia or with sensitivity to even minute quantities of caffeine may find their sleep affected by the green tea flavanols. If this is a problem for you, skip the green tea extract before bed.

Tim recommends taking the supplements six days a week (including your cheat day) and taking one day a week off. In addition, he recommends taking one full week off every two months.

According to *The 4-Hour Body*, these supplements enhance fat loss and speed body recomposition (by storing calories in muscle instead of fat).

Tim also recommends taking a quality B-vitamin supplement while using PAGG.

You can buy each of these supplements separately (and in fact, I do list the names of recommended brands in the Shopping List section.) However, there are more convenient and cost effective options.

The brilliant folks at Pareto Nutrition have developed a custom-blended supplement combination that contains the specific supplements recommended by Tim Ferriss in the correct ratios. Instead of buying five different supplements (PAGG plus the B-vitamin), you can buy the PAGG Stack and get everything you need in two convenient pills: the red pill is for use during the day, and the blue pill is taken at night, before bed. The entire PAGG supplementation is available in a one to six month supplies at a fraction of the cost of buying them separately.

Pareto Nutrition offers continues to research, refine, and tweak their supplement stack to provide the best possible fat-busting formula, and back their product with a money-back guarantee.

Warnings included in 4HB about supplementation specify to use caution if:

• you are undergoing cancer treatment, multiple myeloma or mantle cell lymphoma

• you have any medical conditions such as hypertension, hypoglycemia, diabetes

• you are taking any medications (especially those for blood-thinning, thyroid medications, or anti-anxiety medication.

• you are pregnant or breastfeeding.

In short, use caution and consult with your doctor!

Bingeing (a.k.a. Cheat Day)

The 4-Hour Body advice includes the idea of a cheat or binge day, once per week.

There are multiple purpose for cheat day. It helps with compliance with the rest of the program. You can skip anything, make any changes needed, do whatever it takes, if you know that you just need to make it to Saturday (or whatever day you choose.)

I made a list of everything I wanted, from cookies and ice cream to donuts and pancakes, and ate it all on my cheat day.

The second primary purpose is to keep the body's regulatory mechanisms from decreasing your metabolic rate. With long term dieting, it's likely that your body will slow down its metabolic rate so that you burn less calories. This makes it more difficult to lose weight.

By bingeing once per week, the body's metabolic rate stays high, and you continue to burn calories as though you are not on a diet, leading to faster weight loss.

The Art of Bingeing

Tim recommends three key principles to make the most of your binge. The overall goal is to have as much of the food you eat either be targeted toward muscle building or to pass out of the body without being digested.

#1: Minimize The Release of Insulin

Insulin is a hormone that tells the body to store incoming calories. Tim recommends that the first meal of cheat day should not be crap. It should be high in protein (30 grams) and insoluble fiber (which comes from legumes, aka beans.)

He also recommends consuming a small amount of fructose before the second meal, when your binge starts in earnest. (Ideally this would be a small glass of grapefruit juice, which prolongs the fat-burning effect of coffee.)

Third, use the PAGG supplement combination to increase insulate sensitivity, so that the body will release less insulin.

#2: Increase the Speed of Gastric Emptying

The basic idea is to get the food to pass through your system quickly so that less is digested and more ends up in the toilet.

This sounds strange, but Tim has tested and verified the results. He recommends using caffeine and yerba mate tea, which contains additional stimulants. He has 100-200 milligrams of caffeine or 16 ounces of cooled yerba mate at the biggest binge meals. He also recommends a greens supplement.

#3: Engage in Brief Muscular Contractions Throughout the Binge

According to 4HB, doing 60-120 seconds of brief muscular contractions brings glucose transporter type 4 (aka GLUT-4) to the surface of muscle cells. By comparison, insulin triggers GLUT-4 on fat cells. The more GLUT-4 we have on the surface of muscle cells as opposed to fat cells, the more the body will store incoming nutrients in muscle cells rather than fat cells.

The three recommended exercises are air squats, wall presses, and chest pulls with an elastic band. Do 30 to 50 of two or three of these different exercises before each meal, and optionally again 90 minutes after the meal.

You can find detailed instructions and photographs of each of these exercises on the internet.

For air squats, start by standing straight up. Hold your arms straight out in front of you, parallel to the floor, and with thumbs interlocked. Bend your knees and lower your bottom towards the floor. Your thighs should be parallel with the ground at the bottom. Your arm in front will counter

-balance you to keep you stable. Work up to repeating this 30 to 50 times.

For wall presses, start by standing straight up. Extend your arms out in front of you toward a wall, so that your fully extended arms are 6 to 12 inches from the wall. Keeping your feet where they are, and your body in a straight line, touch the wall with your hands. Now lean into the wall, contracting your arms, until your face almost reaches the wall, then push off again. This is most similar to a pushup against the wall. Work up to repeating 30 to 50 times.

For chest pulls, obtain an elastic band, such as a Theraband. With arms extended, grasp the band about shoulder width apart. Then use your back muscles to extend your arms straight out to the sides, stretching the elastic band. Work up to repeating 30 to 50 times.

Cheat Sheet

Time	Eating Plan	GLUT-4 exercise (optional)	Supplements (optional)	Cold (optional)
Waking				Cold shower, bath, or ice pack for 10 minutes
Just before breakfast		30-50 of each: Air Squats Chest Pulls Wall Presses	AGG	
Breakfast (within 30-60 minutes of waking)	One protein, one legume, one vegetable. 30 grams of protein or more.			
90 minutes after breakfast		*optional: repeat GLUT-4 exercises*		
Just before lunch		30-50 of each: Air Squats Chest Pulls Wall Presses	AGG	
Lunch	One protein, one legume, one vegetable.			
90 minutes after lunch		*optional: repeat GLUT-4 exercises*		
Just before dinner		30-50 of each: Air Squats Chest Pulls Wall Presses	AGG	
Dinner	One protein, one legume, one vegetable.			
90 minutes after dinner		*optional: repeat GLUT-4 exercises*		
Before bedtime			PAG(G)	Cold shower, bath, or ice pack for 10 minutes

Food List	
Proteins	*Egg whites with 1-2 whole eggs, *chicken breast or thigh, beef, fish, pork
Legumes	*Lentils, *black beans, pinto beans, red beans, soybeans
Vegetables	*Spinach, *mixed vegetables (incl. broccoli, cauliflower or other cruciferous), *sauerkraut, *kimchee, peas, green beens, etc.

*Tim says these are associated with the highest rates of fat loss in his experience.

Supplement List	
P: Policosanol	23 mg per day, before bed
A: Alpha-Lipoic Acid (ALA)	300-900 mg per day total, according to schedule.
G: Green Tea Extract	900-1,100 mg per day total, according to schedule. Use decaffeinated extract. According to discussions on popular forums, exclude the Green Tea Extract if it interferes with your sleep, as it does for some people.
G: Garlic	2,000 mg per day total, according to schedule.

Note: 4HB mentions several cautions about supplements, especially for people who are: pregnant, undergoing cancer treatment, taking blood thinning medication, or have any other medical conditions. Please read *The 4-Hour Body* and consult with a doctor.

Cheat Sheet Frequently Asked Questions

After posting the cheat sheet, it was only natural that the questions would start to show up. Here's a few of the most common.

Q: **Am I supposed to have 3 meals or 4 meals per day? The cheat sheet only shows 3, but Tim Ferriss has 4.**

A: Tim Ferriss says you can do either. His guiding advice is to "eat when you're hungry". For many people, 3 meals are more convenient than 4, but if you are consistently getting hungry before your next meal, then it may make sense to do 4 meals. Note that the AGG stack should be taken a maximum of 4 times per day, one of which is at bedtime, so if you do have four meals, don't take AGG with every meal.

Personally, I have two eggs before bed if I'm hungry. This works well for me, and if anything, I seem to notice an increase rate of weight loss.

Q: **Do I have to take a cold shower?**

A: No, the cold shower, the supplements, and the GLUT-4 exercises are all optional. You may lose weight faster, but you should still lose about 15 pounds in the first month just doing the diet portion.

On the other hand, by doing the GLUT-4 exercises (which in total amount to less than 15 minutes of exercise per day) I observed noticeable muscle development and felt stronger.

Q: Do I do the GLUT-4 exercises every day or just on cheat day?

A: The Tim includes the GLUT-4 exercises in the section of *The 4-Hour Body* about binge eating, so the implication is that he is specifically recommending it for cheat days.

However, the basic principle of GLUT-4 exercises is that we can bring GLUT-4 to the surface of muscle cells, and thus have more incoming calories go to muscles instead of fat. This principle works seven days a week. Definitely do the GLUT-4 exercises on cheat day, but also feel free to do them any other time you'd like more muscle development and faster fat loss.

Most people doing the GLUT-4 exercises do them every day.

Q: Do I take PAGG every day or just on cheat day? Do I take Cissus Quad just on cheat day, or every day?

Most people who are following the 4HB and who choose to use PAGG, do so every day. Tim Ferriss does says to skip the PAGG stack one day per week, and one week per month, which suggests that he intends for it to be used on a regular basis, not just cheat day.

However, Cissus Quad is not for long term use, according to Tim. I think he is suggesting that you use it only on cheat day, or for periods of up to four to six weeks.

Q: I am not losing weight, so what am I doing wrong?

A: One possibility is that you're not losing weight because the fat loss is roughly balancing out weight gain. Many people seem to report that their clothes are fitting much better even though they aren't seeing any pounds lost. This is what Tim Ferriss calls body recomposition.

Other likely possibilities include:

- You are making your meals too complex and fancy. Keep it simple, and repeat a few meals.
- You are not eating enough protein. Are you getting at least 30 grams of protein at breakfast, and 20 grams at lunch and dinner? That doesn't mean just 30 grams of food, but actual 30 grams of protein in your food. Not sure? Count your protein for two days.
- See the section "If It's Not Working" later in this book.

I also recommending visiting the 4HB talk forums at http://www.4hbtalk.com/ where many users are helping each other work through these types of problems.

Shopping List

The 4-Hour Body recommends dozen of products. I carefully went through everything in the fat loss section, and put together a consolidated shopping list.

I'm partial to shopping at Amazon for pretty much everything, so links are to the products or closest equivalents that Tim recommends in *The 4-Hour Body* on Amazon. Prices are accurate as of January 3rd, 2011.

You can search for these by name on Amazon by name or access them all online at bit.ly/slowcarbshop.

Measurements
- MyoTape Body Tape Measure ($6.45, equivalent to OrbiTape one handed tape measure.)
- Escali Bio Impedance Scale ($44.95, exact scale recommended by Tim.)
- Slim Guide Skinfold Caliper ($15.65, exact caliper recommended by Tim. Not required to buy both caliper and scale.)

Supplements
- Supercissus Rx Capsules ($26.99, cissus quadrangularis, for use on binge days and periodic supplementation, but not indefinite daily use.)
- Policosanol 23mg, 60 tablets ($24.99, free shipping, part of PAGG)
- Vitamin Shoppe - Alpha-Lipoic Acid, 300 mg ($17.99, 99 cent shipping, part of PAGG)
- Mega Green Tea Extract ($19.24, free shipping, part of PAGG)
- Kyolic Garlic, Formula 100 ($13.50, 99 cent shipping, part of PAGG. Aged garlic.)

- One other item people have been having a hard time finding is the vitamin rich butter, fermented cod liver oil combination recommended by Tim Ferriss. It's not in the fat loss section, but I thought I'd list it here since so many people are looking for it. Blue Ice Royal Butter Oil / Fermented Cod Liver Oil Blend - Capsules is rich in Vitamin K and Vitamin D. Green Pastures is the only supplier of it. They are a family owned farm.

Exercise Equipment

- Thera-band Latex Exercise Bands ($~4.22, free shipping. These are the elastic bands that Tim uses for chest-pulls, the GLUT-4 releasing exercise. Strength varies by color. Small enough to carry in pants pocket.)
- First Place Kettlebells ($60-150. There are many, many kettlebell manufacturers and sellers. This is one 5-star rated kettlebell that is available in a variety of weights. Tim recommends a 20kb/44lb or 24kg/53lb kettlebell for men to start, and a 16kg/35lb or 20kb/44lb kettlebell for women to start.
- I like these no-frills 4.5 star rated Kettlebells that ship free from Amazon: Body-Solid Kettlebells

Meal Plan #1

	Breakfast	Lunch	Dinner	Extra Meal
Sunday	Scrambled eggs w/ spinach, beans of choice	Salmon salad on romaine lettuce	Ground meat, beans, mixed veggies	Fried egg on refried beans
Monday	Fried eggs on refried beans, kimchee on side (3 eggs)	Leftover dinner	Steak, black beans w/ onion, veggies of choice	6-8 brazil nuts
Tuesday	Scrambled eggs w/ spinach, beans of choice	Leftover dinner	Chili: leftover steak & black beans cooked together. Baked broccoli	Egg salad on romaine lettuce
Wednesday	Fried eggs on refried beans, kimchee on side (3 eggs)	Salmon salad on romaine lettuce	OUT: Thai food stir fry, extra veggies instead of rice	Eggs
Thursday	Scrambled eggs w/ spinach, beans of choice	Leftover Thai food	Ground meat, beans, mixed veggies	6-8 brazil nuts
Friday	Scrambled eggs w/ spinach, beans of choice	OUT: Burrito bowl - burrito of choice in bowl, substitute veggies for rice	Leftover dinner	Egg salad on romaine lettuce
Saturday	**Cheat Day! Party like it's 1999!**			

This example meal plan gives you 2 breakfast alternatives, 3 dinner alternatives, and a lunch (which is alternated with leftovers). Included is eating out one lunch a week and one dinner a week. All the meals are (1) exceedingly simple, (2) can meet protein goals, (3) includes protein, beans, and veggies. It's enough variety to keep from going insane, while still having enough repetition to meet the 4 Hour Body fat loss goals. Tips: hot sauce can help reduce gaseousness from eating beans.

Recipes

Scrambled eggs w/ spinach:
Put 1 cup spinach in a medium saute pan, and cook until mostly wilted. Add 3 eggs (2 w/ yolks), and scramble in pan with spinach. Serve with beans of choice, such as refried beans, white kidney beans, or black beans. Cook until done. Cooking time: ~10 minutes.

Salmon Salad on Romaine Lettuce
Buy whole leaf romaine lettuce in supermarket. Open one can of salmon (or tuna if you prefer.) Add about 1-2 tablespoons mayo. If desired, add diced celery. If desired, add wasabi. Mix. Put mixed salmon salad on whole lettuce leaves, like a wrap.
Cooking time: ~5 minutes.

Ground meat, beans, veggies
Saute 1 pound ground meat (beaf, chicken, or turkey) in frying pan, until cooked through, about 7-10 minutes, seasoning with salt, onion, garlic if desired. Place in bowl. Saute frozen mixed veggies package in same pan until done, ~5 minutes. Add to bowl. Saute one can drained beans (cannellini or similar) in frying pan until warm. Add to bowl. Mix contents of bowl. Serve with a little hot sauce if desired. Cooking time: ~20 minutes.

Black beans with onion

Saute onion in pot until cooked. Add canned black beans, bay leaf, garlic and salt seasoning, and simmer gently for ~15 minutes.

Chili

Saute leftover steak for 1 minute (or use cubed raw meat, and saute until browned). Add black beans. Chili seasoning. If desired, diced onion, green peppers, etc.
Cooking time: 10 minutes if using cooked meat, 30-45 minutes if starting with raw meat.

Baked Broccoli

Preheat oven to 425 degrees. Slice broccoli into slabs approximately 1/4 inch thick. Said another way, cut each floret and stem in half the long way. Lightly oil a baking pan, spread broccoli in a single layer. Bake for ten minutes, then turn broccoli over, and bake for ten more minutes. Broccoli will be crisp and slightly browned on the edges. Sprinkle with coarse grained salt.
Cooking time: 5 minutes prep plus 20 minutes cooking.

Meal Plan #2

	Breakfast	Lunch	Dinner	Extra Meal
Sunday	Scrambled eggs w/ mixed frozen veggies, beans of choice	Egg salad on romaine lettuce	Franks and lentils, peas	Two fried eggs
Monday	Huey's Slow Carb Scrambled Eggs	Leftover dinner	BBQ salmon, beans of choice, asparagus	Shot glass (3 TB) of mixed nuts
Tuesday	Fried eggs on refried beans, kimchee on side	Leftover dinner	Crockpot Roast	Hardboiled eggs
Wednesday	Fried eggs on refried beans, guacamole	Leftover dinner	Eat Out: burrito, thai, sashimi, izakaya	More eggs!
Thursday	Scrambled eggs, onions, mushrooms and cannellini beans	Salmon salad on romaine lettuce	Baked chicken, peas, cannellini beans	Shot glass (3 TB) of mixed nuts
Friday		Eat Out: burrito, thai, sashimi, izakaya	Salmon in parchment paper	Tuna salad on romaine lettuce
Saturday	Cheat Day! Party like it's 1999!			

About This Meal Plan

We've added a few seafood dishes and other recipes we'll list below. Also listed are four suggestions for types of food when eating out:

Burrito: In this case, we mean the kind of burrito that is not-a-burrito. Most restaurants will serve your burrito in a bowl without the tortilla. If not, it's not a big deal to just unroll it and eat the insides. Be sure to request no rice, and to substitute with extra veggies if possible.

Thai: Again, there are many thai dishes, such as stir fries that can be slow-carb friendly. Skip the rice. Be careful with curries and spicy dishes, because without the rice as a buffer, these can be tough on your stomach.

Sashimi: Sushi restaurants often serve a sashimi platter that either doesn't include rice, or has the rice on the side. It's just fish and daikon radish, usually. Edamame and seaweed salad are other good choices here.

Izakaya: Izakaya are Japanese restaurants that specialize in food accompaniments to drinking. That's a fancy way of saying bar food. What you'll find here are meat skewers, japanese pickles, vegetables, and more.

Recipes

Egg Salad

1. Hard boil 3 eggs. (Place eggs in cold water on stove. Turn temperature to high. When water boils, turn temperature down low, and start timer. At 12 minutes, take eggs out and plunge into icy-cold water. Immediately break eggs and leave in cold water for 1 minute more. Remove and peel shells.)
2. Put peeled eggs in bowl. Using tines of fork, crush eggs until mixture is crumble. Add about a tablespoon

of mayonnaise, a teaspoon of mustard, salt and pepper to taste.

3. If serving on romaine lettuce, get whole romaine lettuce heads from the grocery. Peel off 3 or 4 lettuce leaves, rinse and dry. Spoon the egg salad into the leaves, and eat like a burrito.

Huey's Slow Carb Scrambled Egg Breakfast

This recipe is from Huey Davis at litelifestyle.com, via Tim Ferriss's Slow Carb Cookbook.

Ingredients:
1/2 can of black beans
2 medium eggs
2 Tbsp of medium chunky salsa
1/2 Haas avocado

1. Place the black beans in a pan and set to low heat.
2. Break the two eggs in a bowl, add a splash of water, and beat them with a fork.
3. Heat a frying pan on medium heat with some vegetable oil.
4. When the pan is ready, cook the eggs until there is no liquid visible.
5. Pour the scrambled eggs and black beans onto a plate.
6. Add the two Tbsp of salsa to the eggs, and the half of avocado. Enjoy!

BBQ Salmon

1. Get fresh, wild-caught salmon from your local supermarket. (My personal recommendation is to avoid farmed salmon. Just Google "farmed salmon".)
2. Using a baking pan of sufficient size to hold the salmon, pour in about 1/2 cup olive oil, 1/2 cup soy

sauce. (Over time, adjust for the size of fish you have.) Add a tablespoon of honey, and a teaspoon of wasabi. (OK, we're cheating here with the honey, but just a wee little bit.) Mix ingredients with fork until blended.

3. Lay salmon in pan on mixture, skin side up, for at least 30 minutes. (You can do this in the fridge, and you can do it for longer if you want.)
4. Preheat BBQ.
5. Place salmon on BBQ, medium-high heat.
6. Check the salmon at about five minutes, and then every minute or two after that, until done. Signs that it is done:
   - You'll start to see white lines on the surface, where some of the fat comes out.
   - You push apart the flakes of salmon, and the fish is opaque, not translucent.
   Some like their fish completely opaque. I prefer it to be about two thirds opaque.
7. Remove from grill and serve immediately.

Scrambled eggs, onions, mushrooms

1. Dice 1/2 onion and 4 shiitake mushrooms into 1/2 inch pieces. (shiitake mushrooms are supposed to have immune boosting properties, but of course you could do this with another kind of mushroom.)
2. Heat 1 TB of olive oil in frying pan over medium heat. Saute onion and mushrooms, stirring frequently.
3. Meanwhile, scramble 3 eggs in a bowl with a fork.
4. If necessary, add a little butter or oil to the frying pan, if it appears dry, then pour in the eggs. Stir every 20 seconds or so, until done. Done varying by preference: some prefer their eggs slightly wet, while others like them completely dry.

Salmon in Parchment Paper

This dish, known as Poisson en Papillate (Fish in Parchment Paper), is fun and delicious.

Using parchment paper to cook the fish allows the fish to retain all of its natural juices and infuses it with the flavors of the accompanying vegetables and herbs. It should also puff up slightly, making a nice presentation for the table.

Parchment paper can be found in most groceries stores. (It is not the same thing as wax paper.) Don't be overwhelmed by the number of ingredients. Just prep the ingredients first, then assemble.

Ingredients:
4 pieces (15" x 11" approx.) parchment paper
1 cup carrot, diced
4 4 oz salmons fillets (also works great with halibut, cod, snapper)
salt and freshly ground pepper
8 sprigs fresh thyme
1 shallot, finely minced
1 tbsp fresh lemon juice
1/2 cup leeks (white and pale green part only), thinly sliced
1/2 cup mushrooms, sliced
2 tbsp dry white wine
4 tsp butter
2 tbsp fresh parsley, chopped

Preheat oven to 450 degrees. On one piece parchment paper, place 1/4 cup carrots in center, and top with a fish fillet. Season with salt and pepper. Top fillet with 2 sprigs thyme, and 1/4 of the shallot, lemon juice, leeks, mushrooms, and wine. Top with 1 tsp butter and season with a little more salt and pepper.

Draw up the two long edges of paper together, and fold over several times. Then take each end, one at a time, and fold up and over several times. Secure, using either staples, paperclip, or twine.

The whole package should hold in the liquids you added plus the natural juices of the fish, and it should seem nearly airtight. If so, then repeat for for the remaining fish fillets.

Carefully place packages on baking sheet and place in oven. Bake 12 minutes or until package puffs up and fish flakes easily with a fork. Thick fish fillets will take longer - from 15 to 18 minutes - but be sure to check one around 12 minutes to avoid overcooking.

Transfer packages to plates and cut up at the table. Be careful of hot steam when opening. Sprinkle with parsley and enjoy.

Will's Indian Style Franks and Lentils

This is one of my favorite recipes - it's simple, inexpensive, and very tasty. The only thing Indian style about this is the choice of primary seasonings (cumin and turmeric) and beans (lentils). It just makes for a good name. This makes enough for about eight large servings:

Ingredients:
1.5 cups of brown lentils
5 cups of water
1 bullion cube
generous sprinkling of cumin (1/4 teaspoon)
very generous sprinkling of turmeric (1/2 teaspoon)
1 to 3 Country Natural Beef hot dogs or other natural, smoky hot dog
1/2 to 1 onion, diced (optional)
assorted vegetables or greens, such as carrots, spinach, swiss chard, etc. (optional)

Country Natural Beef hot dogs are a particular brand of all natural beef hot dogs available in natural food stores on the West Coast. They have a wonderful smoky flavor that adds substantially to the this dish. I've tried substitutes, but the result was never as good. The franks are important for the flavor of the dish, but the quantity can be adjusted to suit your budget and desire.

Wash the lentils, add water, bullion cube, spices, and optional onion, and bring to a boil. Cover and cook for 35-45 minutes. Add hot dogs at the 15 minute mark. Add other vegetables and greens after a suitable amount of time: carrots should cook for about 10-15 minutes, greens for only a minute or two, etc.

If you like a mild spicy flavor, I highly recommend The Wizard's Organic Hot Stuff Piquante Sauce, which seems to complement the other flavors in this dish very well. Or a sprinkling of cayenne powder after cooking is good if you're looking for straight up spiciness.

Effectiveness of Slow Carb / Fat Loss Regimen

I started reading *The 4-Hour Body* by Tim Ferris on Christmas day, and by two days later, I had started the fat loss program. By day 28, I stopped to keep track of my findings. Here's what I discovered:

Tim says you can lose 20 pounds of fat in 28 days, while gaining 5 pounds of muscle for a net loss of 15 pounds of weight. So 28 days has passed. How did I do?

I lost 13.6 pounds in 28 days, going from 205 to 191.4. I lost 5.5 total inches (sum of circumference of biceps, thighs, hips, and navel). I'm using a bioimpedence scale to measure body fat, which is not the most accurate tool, but I did follow Tim's suggestion of having two glasses of cold water on waking, and measuring 20 minutes later. I only obtained the scale two weeks in. I saw my body fat drop 0.8% in two weeks. In sum, I would consider this a good success.

For four straight days in week three, due to work stress and other events, I cheated on the diet, and saw myself gain back 2.5 pounds. Had I stuck with it through those days, I believe I would have easily hit the 15-pounds that Tim said would be possible.

Those are the numbers. Now let me give you the experiential perspective:

Week 1:

I start the fat loss program. The key elements are that I'm not allowed to have any grains or sugars, except on one cheat day per week. (There are other restrictions, such as no dairy, that don't affect me because I didn't eat dairy.) Meals consist of a protein source, a legume, and vegetables. I enjoy the food very much (I love beans), but I'm shocked by how much protein I have to eat. It takes about 3 days before I'm eating enough protein for breakfast (target: 30 grams of net protein.) Meals can be as big as I want, and I eat enough to make sure I won't be hungry before the next meal.

I find that I really miss my snacks. I find myself in the kitchen at least once every 30 minutes looking for a snack even though I don't feel hungry.

It's hard to stick it out. I concede and allow myself 4 nuts in the afternoon and 4 nuts in the evening as a pure "snack" food. I continue this practice for all 28 days.

I also continue my practice of having a drink every evening, even though this is not strictly part of the diet.

I notice that sinus congestion, a chronic condition I am used to dealing with, goes away almost completely, probably due to removing grains from my diet.

Favorite meal of the week: salmon salad on whole romaine lettuce leaves.

I go from 205 to a low of 197, then enjoy my cheat day. I pig out, eating an entire tray of honey cookies that could normally feed about 8 people, 2 bowls of ice cream, 4 bowls of potato chips, 3 bowls of pretzels, 2 bowls of nuts, and a large number of chocolate candies.

Week 2:

I am actually relieved to get back to the diet after making myself slightly sick on cheat day.

Cravings for snacks continue, although the number of times per day I find myself in the kitchen goes down slightly.

I am back at work in my office, and find it's very boring to go through a whole day of work without snacks. I relish in the fact that coffee is still allowed, and even encouraged as it helps fat loss.

I start GLUT-4 exercises, and enjoy using the Theraband Latex Exercise Bands. It feels good to be doing something other than just sitting in front of the computer.

I start using the supplements that Tim recommends.

I start cold showers this week, another tactic that Tim encourages to help the body burn fat, and start noticing a correlation between high weight loss days and the cold showers.

I start this week at 200 (I make it a policy not to weigh myself on the day after cheat day), and hit a low of 195.6, a loss of 1.4 pounds over my previous week low.

Week 3:

Cravings for snacks diminishes this week, and yet strangely this is my hardest week yet. I end up cheating on the diet on 4 consecutive days. All of these behaviors I would attribute to stress. Only one of these is my official cheat day, and the other days I only have "small" snacks: a chocolate candy or a cookie. Yet I see my weight loss completely stall on these days.

I start the week at 196.2 and hit a low of 193.8, a loss of 1.8 pounds over my previous week low.

Week 4:

Cravings for snacks is at it's lowest. I stick to the diet for the whole week. When I have any intense stress related cravings, I get myself a cup of no-calorie chocolate tea, which smells great and is oddly satisfying.

I start kettlebell exercises.

I start the week at 196.8 and hit a low of 191.4, a loss of 2.4 pounds of my previous week low. I've gone from 205 to 191.4 in 25 days.

Summary

I feel like this is something I can easily stick with as long as necessary. I don't feel hungry, I don't have to count calories, and I have an allocated day to being able to eat anything I can. Compliance is easy, and it's clearly effective as I'm losing weight steadily.

Fifteen Months Later

The above was written just 28 days after starting the fat loss regimen. I continued to follow the slow carb diet and the fat loss recommendations for more than fifteen months, continuing up to the present day.

At the end of twelve months I had lost twenty pounds (going from 205 originally to 185). In the first few months of the following year I lost another five pounds, bringing me to a total of twenty-five pounds lost and an end weight of 180. As I'm a six foot tall male, I'm pretty close to my ideal weight.

I continue to follow the program to maintain my weight and because I believe the diet is healthier than my old ways of eating, which involved too much sugar and refined grains.

I may have two cheat days a week, or even occasionally an entire week or two where I lapse, but most of the time I stick to the slow carb program as Tim explained it: legumes, vegetables, and protein at every meal, and no sugars or starches.

Why Calories-In/Calories-Out is a Fallacy

It's been fascinating to see how The 4 Hour Body has provoked arguments and disparaging comments in virtually every online fitness community. Typically it looks something like this:

- Original poster: Hi, I am trying Tim Ferriss's fat loss program in The 4 Hour Body, and I am losing a lot of weight. It's great. What have been other people's experiences?
- Response #1: weight loss is a simple matter of calories-in, calories-out. If you want to lose weight, you take in less calories, or put out more calories. I don't need to spend $14 to learn that.
- Response #2: Who are you to be posting in our community? I've never seen you post here before.
- Response #3: What is it with all these people posting about The 4 Hour Body? I think Tim Ferriss must be paying people to go around posting.

I saw this happen in half dozen other communities. As someone who understands online communities, and as someone who is new to fitness via The 4 Hour Body, I think it's an interesting issue to observe.

Here's what I see happening:

Someone who has not been into fitness, perhaps because they haven't had success with diets or exercise programs before, tries The 4-Hour Body and has success. They get excited and want to share their experience.

The established community sees a bunch of newcomers spouting off counter-intuitive fitness information, may have heard some controversy about Tim Ferriss or the 4

Hour Body, and so they reject the new community members summarily.

The same thing can happen on a lesser scale in the real-world when you share your success with friends and family. The information may seem so contradictory to "common sense" that it is rejected.

I want to address just one part of the conflict, because it's typically the first issue raised: the established community or friends and family says something to the effect of: "Weight loss is simple, you either reduce calories in, or you increase calories-out." That's what they say, but what I think they mean is closer to: "You either restrict the quantity you eat or you exercise more." It sounds like they want you to suffer, you just get to pick the form of suffering.

There's two reasons why this statement is in conflict with the principles of The 4 Hour Body:

1. The 4 Hour Body fat loss program doesn't require restricting food intake. In fact, Tim says, "If you're hungry, eat more."

2. The 4 Hour Body fat loss program doesn't require people to spend time exercising, although you can optionally do 5 minutes of exercises before each meal for more rapid results. But 5 minutes of exercises is not the same kind of burden as taking an hour or two out of your day to exercise and shower.

Here are just a few of the differences:

The 4HB fat loss section emphasizes eating more protein, and no grains, sugars, or fruits. Protein itself has less available calories (3.2/gram) than is normally listed as (4.0/gram), and so it's already a win over carbohydrates.

On top of that, the body directly excretes up to 1/3 of excess protein that can't be used, whereas the equivalent in carbs would be more efficiently converted to fat.

By ensuring that people eat higher quality foods (protein, legumes, vegetables), they have more energy, and can more easily cut the snacking cycle. This may indeed reduce calories-in greatly, but it's vastly different than just telling people to "eat less."

The use of a high protein diet stimulates metabolism, increasing calories-out without the use of exercise.

Similarly, cold therapy stimulates metabolism and increases calories-out without the use of exercise.

GLUT-4 exercises (2-3 minutes of fast paced exercises) redirects incoming calories to muscle development rather than being stored away as fat, a term that Tim calls body recomposition. It is far easier to do and to sustain a few minutes of exercise before a meal compared to taking 60-90 minutes out of your day to "go exercise", and so most people wouldn't consider this as exercise per say.

If It's Not Working

After my blog posts on *The 4-Hour Body*, I started
receiving emails from readers. About 1 in 10 would tell me
that the 4HB didn't seem to be working for them.

They reporting doing the slow-carb diet, the GLUT4
exercises, taking the PAGG stack, and not losing weight. I've
seen similar stories on other 4 Hour Body forums.

Here are a few thoughts:

Even among many people who are not losing weight
on the scale, they suddenly find their clothes are fitting better.
Tim Ferriss calls this body recomposition, and he even says
in the 4HB that you may lose 20 pounds of fat, but gain 5
pounds of muscle.

I wonder if, for some people, this principle may be
happening in extreme. Perhaps they are putting on lots of
muscle. They may not see a net loss of weight, but they look
and feel better. Instead of measuring pounds only, measure
total inches, body-fat percentage, and take those full body
photos to see if the diet really is having an effect.

Tim Ferriss has noted, on the Amazon Q&A page for
The 4-Hour Body, women will be less likely to notice significant
weight loss during the first few weeks, although they will
notice body recomposition effects. He says the weight loss
will kick in around weeks 3-4.

I've noticed that some of the people who aren't losing
weight write extensively about the amount of beans and
vegetables they are eating, but don't mention anything about
protein. Conversely, there's another group that write
extensively about the protein shakes they are consuming.

For both of these groups may do better to focus on
real-food protein. Eat eggs, fish, and meat to get 30 grams or
more of protein at breakfast, and 20 grams or more of protein

at lunch and dinner. Don't do protein shakes and don't obsess over beans and veggies. Protein shakes in particular are tricky, because most include carbs, and because the protein they contain is processed, which changes the way the body processes it.

If you must do protein shakes, I've seen Tim Ferriss recommend unflavored whey protein shakes on the Amazon question and answer boards.

Watch out for the snack foods. At Tim says, any food that you can't consume just one of is a risk. So nuts, jerky, or even beans are all foods that may be part of the diet, but you can eat them mindlessly. Don't do that. Eat meals. If you get too hungry with three meals, then eat four, but don't snack.

Visit the 4HB Talk forums[2], where many other people like you are sharing their experiences and working through these issues.

---

[2] http://4hbtalk.com

Taking a Cold Shower

If you've been reading *The 4-Hour Body*, then you probably know that one of the techniques Tim recommends that can help you lose fat faster is to take cold showers. Cold showers burn fat in several ways:

- They stimulate your brown fat cells, helping the ones you have reproduce, work harder.
- They cause your body to compensate for the loss of body heat through shivering and a higher metabolic rate.
- But cold showers have many other benefits as well:
- They can help reduce or avoid depression.
- Improves circulation, which is good for overall cardiac health.
- Strengthens your immune system.
- Increases testosterone and fertility.
- Heck, even James Bond takes cold showers.

But how do you take a cold shower? If you just jump into cold water, you'll be miserable. There's a good technique that minimize the unpleasantness and actually maximizes the benefit you'll get, because you'll be able to stick with it better.

1. Start with a normal, hot shower.
2. Shampoo your hair and rinse normally.
3. Soap up in the hot water.
4. Then, turn the temperature to a low luke-warm. Nothing that you'd identify as cold, just neither cold nor warm.
5. Rinse off in this low luke-warm water. This gives your body time to adjust to the temperature.
6. Now, turn your back to the water.
7. Turn the temperature down slightly, just a few degrees cooler.

8. Wait about 30-40 seconds. You can count off one-one thousand, two-one thousand, or you can sing the ABCs.
9. Repeat 7 and 8, as many times as you can. I can now go about 6 cycles of gradually reducing the temperature.

I usually stop the cycle after my teeth start chattering while singing the ABCs.

The reason this process works is:
- You still get to enjoy a hot shower to start.
- You gradually reduce the temperature so that it is never an unpleasant shock.
- By the time the water temperature is getting really cold, your upper back and neck are already somewhat numb, so you hardly notice the temperature change.

Using this method, you should easily be able to spend 5-6 minutes in an increasingly cold shower. You'll finish feeling invigorated and refreshed. Give it a try!

Cut Outs

Following this page you'll find copies of the cheat sheet, the supplement and food list charts, and the meal plans.

Cut these out and place them on your fridge, office wall, or where ever they will help you.

4-Hour Body Cheat Sheet				
Time	Eating Plan	GLUT-4 exercise (optional)	Supplements (optional)	Cold (optional)
Waking				Cold shower, bath, or ice pack for 10 minutes
Just before breakfast		30-50 of each: Air Squats Chest Pulls Wall Presses	AGG	
Breakfast (within 30-60 minutes of waking)	One protein, one legume, one vegetable. 30 grams of protein or more.			
90 minutes after breakfast		optional: repeat GLUT-4 exercises		
Just before lunch		30-50 of each: Air Squats Chest Pulls Wall Presses	AGG	
Lunch	One protein, one legume, one vegetable.			
90 minutes after lunch		optional: repeat GLUT-4 exercises		
Just before dinner		30-50 of each: Air Squats Chest Pulls Wall Presses	AGG	
Dinner	One protein, one legume, one vegetable.			
90 minutes after dinner		optional: repeat GLUT-4 exercises		
Before bedtime			PAG(G)	Cold shower, bath, or ice pack for 10 minutes

Food List	
Proteins	*Egg whites with 1-2 whole eggs, *chicken breast or thigh, beef, fish, pork
Legumes	*Lentils, *black beans, pinto beans, red beans, soybeans
Vegetables	*Spinach, *mixed vegetables (incl. broccoli, cauliflower or other cruciferous), *sauerkraut, *kimchee, peas, green beens, etc.

Supplement List	
P: Policosanol	23 mg per day, before bed
A: Alpha-lipoic Acid (ALA)	300-900 mg per day total, according to schedule.
G: Green Tea Extract	900-1,100 mg per day total, according to schedule. Use decaffeinated extract. According to discussions on popular forums, exclude the Green Tea Extract if it interferes with your sleep, as it does for some people.
G: Garlic	2,000 mg per day total, according to schedule.

Meal Plan #1	Breakfast	Lunch	Dinner	Extra Meal
Sunday	Scrambled eggs w/ spinach, beans of choice	Salmon salad on romaine lettuce	Ground meat, beans, mixed veggies	Fried egg on refried beans
Monday	Fried eggs on refried beans, kimchee on side (3 eggs)	Leftover dinner	Steak, black beans w/ onion, veggies of choice	6-8 brazil nuts
Tuesday	Scrambled eggs w/ spinach, beans of choice	Leftover dinner	Chili: leftover steak & black beans cooked together. Baked broccoli	Egg salad on romaine lettuce
Wednesday	Fried eggs on refried beans, kimchee on side (3 eggs)	Salmon salad on romaine lettuce	OUT: Thai food stir fry, extra veggies instead of rice	Eggs
Thursday	Scrambled eggs w/ spinach, beans of choice	Leftover Thai food	Ground meat, beans, mixed veggies	6-8 brazil nuts
Friday	Scrambled eggs w/ spinach, beans of choice	OUT: Burrito bowl - burrito of choice in bowl, substitute veggies for rice	Leftover dinner	Egg salad on romaine lettuce
Saturday	Cheat Day! Party like it's 1999!			

51

Meal Plan #2	Breakfast	Lunch	Dinner	Extra Meal
Sunday	Scrambled eggs w/ mixed frozen veggies, beans of choice	Egg salad on romaine lettuce	Franks and lentils, peas	Two fried eggs
Monday	Huey's Slow Carb Scrambled Eggs	Leftover dinner	BBQ salmon, beans of choice, asparagus	Shot glass (3 TB) of mixed nuts
Tuesday	Fried eggs on refried beans, kimchee on side	Leftover dinner	Crockpot Roast	Hardboiled eggs
Wednesday	Fried eggs on refried beans, guacamole	Leftover dinner	Eat Out: burrito, thai, sashimi, izakaya	More eggs!
Thursday	Scrambled eggs, onions, mushrooms and cannellini beans	Salmon salad on romaine lettuce	Baked chicken, peas, cannellini beans	Shot glass (3 TB) of mixed nuts
Friday		Eat Out: burrito, thai, sashimi, izakaya	Salmon in parchment paper	Tuna salad on romaine lettuce
Saturday	Cheat Day! Party like it's 1999!			

Food List

Proteins	*Egg whites with 1-2 whole eggs, *chicken breast or thigh, beef, fish, pork
Legumes	*Lentils, *black beans, pinto beans, red beans, soybeans
Vegetables	*Spinach, *mixed vegetables (incl. broccoli, cauliflower or other cruciferous), *sauerkraut, *kimchee, peas, green beens, etc.

Supplement List

P: Policosanol	23 mg per day, before bed
A: Alpha-lipoic Acid (ALA)	300-900 mg per day total, according to schedule.
G: Green Tea Extract	900-1,100 mg per day total, according to schedule. Use decaffeinated extract. According to discussions on popular forums, exclude the Green Tea Extract if it interferes with your sleep, as it does for some people.
G: Garlic	2,000 mg per day total, according to schedule.

4-Hour Body Cheat Sheet

Time	Eating Plan	GLUT-4 exercise (optional)	Supplements (optional)	Cold (optional)
Waking				Cold shower, bath, or ice pack for 10 minutes
Just before breakfast		30-50 of each: Air Squats Chest Pulls Wall Presses	AGG	
Breakfast (within 30-60 minutes of waking)	One protein, one legume, one vegetable. 30 grams of protein or more.			
90 minutes after breakfast		optional: repeat GLUT-4 exercises		
Just before lunch		30-50 of each: Air Squats Chest Pulls Wall Presses	AGG	
Lunch	One protein, one legume, one vegetable.			
90 minutes after lunch		optional: repeat GLUT-4 exercises		
Just before dinner		30-50 of each: Air Squats Chest Pulls Wall Presses	AGG	
Dinner	One protein, one legume, one vegetable.			
90 minutes after dinner		optional: repeat GLUT-4 exercises		
Before bedtime			PAG(G)	Cold shower, bath, or ice pack for 10 minutes

Meal Plan #1

Meal Plan #1	Breakfast	Lunch	Dinner	Extra Meal
Sunday	Scrambled eggs w/ spinach, beans of choice	Salmon salad on romaine lettuce	Ground meat, beans, mixed veggies	Fried egg on refried beans
Monday	Fried eggs on refried beans	Leftover dinner	Steak, black beans w/ onion, veggies of choice	6-8 brazil nuts
Tuesday	Scrambled eggs w/ spinach, beans of choice	Leftover dinner	Chili: leftover steak & black beans cooked together. Baked broccoli.	Egg salad on romaine lettuce
Wednesday	Fried eggs on refried beans, kimchee on side (3 eggs)	Salmon salad on romaine lettuce	OUT: Thai food stir fry, extra veggies instead of rice	Eggs
Thursday	Scrambled eggs w/ spinach, beans of choice	Leftover Thai food	Ground meat, beans, mixed veggies	6-8 brazil nuts
Friday	Scrambled eggs w/ spinach, beans of choice	OUT: Burrito bowl - burrito of choice in bowl, substitute veggies for rice	Leftover dinner	Egg salad on romaine lettuce
Saturday	Cheat Day! Party like it's 1999!			

Meal Plan #2

Meal Plan #2	Breakfast	Lunch	Dinner	Extra Meal
Sunday	Scrambled eggs w/ mixed frozen veggies, beans of choice	Egg salad on romaine lettuce	Franks and lentils, peas	Two fried eggs
Monday	Huey's Slow Carb Scrambled Eggs	Leftover dinner	BBQ salmon, beans of choice, asparagus	Shot glass (3 TB) of mixed nuts
Tuesday	Fried eggs on refried beans, kimchee on side	Leftover dinner	Crockpot Roast	Hardboiled eggs
Wednesday	Fried eggs on refried beans, guacamole	Leftover dinner	Eat Out: burrito, thai, sashimi, izakaya	More eggs!
Thursday	Scrambled eggs, onions, mushrooms and cannellini beans	Salmon salad on romaine lettuce	Baked chicken, peas, cannellini beans	Shot glass (3 TB) of mixed nuts
Friday		Eat Out: burrito, thai, sashimi, izakaya	Salmon in parchment paper	Tuna salad on romaine lettuce
Saturday	Cheat Day! Party like it's 1999!			

Acknowledgements

I want to start by thanking Tim Ferriss for researching and writing *The 4-Hour Body*. I continue to be inspired and learn new things every time I open it up.

I also want to thank Jason Glaspey, founder of paleoplan.com, for the inspiration to publish this book.

Thanks to the many readers of my blog who gave feedback on articles, asked questions, pushed for improvements, and keep the conversation lively.

Finally, thanks to my friends and family for their ongoing support. I couldn't do it without you.

William Hertling

23415790R00039

Made in the USA
San Bernardino, CA
18 August 2015